THIS BBQ JOURNAL

Belongs to...

_____

DEDICATION

This book is dedicated to all the grill masters out there who love to start up the grill and create a masterpiece.

You are my inspiration for producing books
and I'm honored to be a part of keeping your grilling and smoking experiences organized.

This journal notebook will help you record your details and experience while you grill.

Thoughtfully put together with these sections to record, Date, The Meat, The Prep, Grill/Cooker, Technique and Results.

I hope you enjoy each and every masterpiece you create while you document your process!

HOW TO USE THIS BOOK:

The purpose of this book is to keep all of your grilling and smoking experiences and findings all in one place. It will help keep you organized.

This BBQ Journal Log will allow you to accurately document all the things you want to remember about your experience of grilling and smoking. It's a great way to chart your course through the world of meat.

Here are examples of the prompts for you to fill in and write about your experience and findings in this book:

1. Date - Record the day and date of your barbecue.
2. The Meat - Write in the Cut, Price, Source, Weight, Expiration Date, Fresh/ Frozen, Notes.
3. The Prep - Log the Wood Flavor, Soaked/ Dry, Wood Type, Quantity, Rub/ Marinade/ Seasoning/ Brine, Mop/ Paste/ Sauce.
4. Grill/ Cooker - Cooker used, Blank Lined Notes
5. Technique - For writing the Time, Cooker Target Temp, Cooker Actual Temp, Meat Temp, Weather Temp, Actions Taken (Vents, Wood, Mop or Turn).
6. Results - Write Notes & Serving & Rate your results 1-10.

Let's get smoking!

Date

The Meat

Cut	Price
Source	Weight
Expiration Date	Fresh/Frozen

Notes

The Prep

Wood Flavour	Soaked/Dry
Wood type	Quantity

Rub/Marinade/Seasoning/Brine

Mop/Paste/Sauce

It's smoking time...

Cooker used

Notes

Log all that deliciousness...

Time	Cooker Target Temp	Cooker Actual Temp	Meat Temp	Weather Temp	Action taken e.g. vents, wood, mop or turn

Results

RATING	1	2	3	4	5	6	7	8	9	10

Notes/serving

Let's get smoking!

Date

The Meat

Cut		Price	
Source		Weight	
Expiration Date		Fresh/Frozen	
Notes			

The Prep

Wood Flavour		Soaked/Dry	
Wood type		Quantity	
Rub/Marinade/Seasoning/Brine			
Mop/Paste/Sauce			

It's smoking time...

Cooker used
Notes

Log all that deliciousness...

Time	Cooker Target Temp	Cooker Actual Temp	Meat Temp	Weather Temp	Action taken e.g. vents, wood, mop or turn

Results

RATING   1   2   3   4   5   6   7   8   9   10

Notes/serving

Let's get smoking!

Date

The Meat

Cut		Price	
Source		Weight	
Expiration Date		Fresh/Frozen	

Notes

The Prep

Wood Flavour		Soaked/Dry	
Wood type		Quantity	

Rub/Marinade/Seasoning/Brine

Mop/Paste/Sauce

It's smoking time...

Cooker used

Notes

Log all that deliciousness...

Time	Cooker Target Temp	Cooker Actual Temp	Meat Temp	Weather Temp	Action taken e.g. vents, wood, mop or turn

Results

RATING	1	2	3	4	5	6	7	8	9	10

Notes/serving

Let's get smoking!

Date

The Meat

Cut		Price	
Source		Weight	
Expiration Date		Fresh/Frozen	
Notes			

The Prep

Wood Flavour		Soaked/Dry	
Wood type		Quantity	
Rub/Marinade/Seasoning/Brine			
Mop/Paste/Sauce			

It's smoking time...

Cooker used
Notes

Log all that deliciousness...

Time	Cooker Target Temp	Cooker Actual Temp	Meat Temp	Weather Temp	Action taken e.g. vents, wood, mop or turn

Results

RATING	1	2	3	4	5	6	7	8	9	10

Notes/serving

Let's get smoking!

Date

The Meat

Cut	Price
Source	Weight
Expiration Date	Fresh/Frozen
Notes	

The Prep

Wood Flavour	Soaked/Dry
Wood type	Quantity
Rub/Marinade/Seasoning/Brine	
Mop/Paste/Sauce	

It's smoking time...

Cooker used
Notes

Log all that deliciousness...

Time	Cooker Target Temp	Cooker Actual Temp	Meat Temp	Weather Temp	Action taken e.g. vents, wood, mop or turn

Results

RATING   1   2   3   4   5   6   7   8   9   10

Notes/serving

Let's get smoking!

Date

The Meat

Cut	Price
Source	Weight
Expiration Date	Fresh/Frozen
Notes	

The Prep

Wood Flavour	Soaked/Dry
Wood type	Quantity
Rub/Marinade/Seasoning/Brine	
Mop/Paste/Sauce	

It's smoking time...

Cooker used
Notes

Log all that deliciousness...

Time	Cooker Target Temp	Cooker Actual Temp	Meat Temp	Weather Temp	Action taken e.g. vents, wood, mop or turn

Results

RATING	1	2	3	4	5	6	7	8	9	10

Notes/serving

Let's get smoking!

Date

The Meat

Cut	Price
Source	Weight
Expiration Date	Fresh/Frozen

Notes

The Prep

Wood Flavour	Soaked/Dry
Wood type	Quantity

Rub/Marinade/Seasoning/Brine

Mop/Paste/Sauce

It's smoking time...

Cooker used

Notes

Log all that deliciousness...

Time	Cooker Target Temp	Cooker Actual Temp	Meat Temp	Weather Temp	Action taken e.g. vents, wood, mop or turn

Results

RATING 1   2   3   4   5   6   7   8   9   10

Notes/serving

Let's get smoking!

Date

The Meat

Cut		Price	
Source		Weight	
Expiration Date		Fresh/Frozen	
Notes			

The Prep

Wood Flavour		Soaked/Dry	
Wood type		Quantity	
Rub/Marinade/Seasoning/Brine			
Mop/Paste/Sauce			

It's smoking time...

Cooker used
Notes

Log all that deliciousness...

Time	Cooker Target Temp	Cooker Actual Temp	Meat Temp	Weather Temp	Action taken e.g. vents, wood, mop or turn

Results

RATING   1   2   3   4   5   6   7   8   9   10

Notes/serving

Let's get smoking!

Date

The Meat

Cut	Price
Source	Weight
Expiration Date	Fresh/Frozen

Notes

The Prep

Wood Flavour	Soaked/Dry
Wood type	Quantity

Rub/Marinade/Seasoning/Brine

Mop/Paste/Sauce

It's smoking time...

Cooker used

Notes

Log all that deliciousness...

Time	Cooker Target Temp	Cooker Actual Temp	Meat Temp	Weather Temp	Action taken e.g. vents, wood, mop or turn

Results

RATING   1   2   3   4   5   6   7   8   9   10

Notes/serving

Let's get smoking!

Date

The Meat

Cut	Price
Source	Weight
Expiration Date	Fresh/Frozen

Notes

The Prep

Wood Flavour	Soaked/Dry
Wood type	Quantity

Rub/Marinade/Seasoning/Brine

Mop/Paste/Sauce

It's smoking time...

Cooker used

Notes

Log all that deliciousness...

Time	Cooker Target Temp	Cooker Actual Temp	Meat Temp	Weather Temp	Action taken e.g. vents, wood, mop or turn

Results

RATING	1	2	3	4	5	6	7	8	9	10

Notes/serving

Let's get smoking!

Date

The Meat

Cut	Price
Source	Weight
Expiration Date	Fresh/Frozen

Notes

The Prep

Wood Flavour	Soaked/Dry
Wood type	Quantity

Rub/Marinade/Seasoning/Brine

Mop/Paste/Sauce

It's smoking time...

Cooker used

Notes

Log all that deliciousness...

Time	Cooker Target Temp	Cooker Actual Temp	Meat Temp	Weather Temp	Action taken e.g. vents, wood, mop or turn

Results

RATING   1   2   3   4   5   6   7   8   9   10

Notes/serving

Let's get smoking!

Date

The Meat

Cut	Price
Source	Weight
Expiration Date	Fresh/Frozen

Notes

The Prep

Wood Flavour	Soaked/Dry
Wood type	Quantity

Rub/Marinade/Seasoning/Brine

Mop/Paste/Sauce

It's smoking time...

Cooker used

Notes

Log all that deliciousness...

Time	Cooker Target Temp	Cooker Actual Temp	Meat Temp	Weather Temp	Action taken e.g. vents, wood, mop or turn

Results

RATING   1   2   3   4   5   6   7   8   9   10

Notes/serving

Let's get smoking!

Date

The Meat

Cut	Price
Source	Weight
Expiration Date	Fresh/Frozen

Notes

The Prep

Wood Flavour	Soaked/Dry
Wood type	Quantity

Rub/Marinade/Seasoning/Brine

Mop/Paste/Sauce

It's smoking time...

Cooker used

Notes

Log all that deliciousness...

Time	Cooker Target Temp	Cooker Actual Temp	Meat Temp	Weather Temp	Action taken e.g. vents, wood, mop or turn

Results

RATING	1	2	3	4	5	6	7	8	9	10

Notes/serving

Let's get smoking!

Date

The Meat

Cut	Price
Source	Weight
Expiration Date	Fresh/Frozen

Notes

The Prep

Wood Flavour	Soaked/Dry
Wood type	Quantity

Rub/Marinade/Seasoning/Brine

Mop/Paste/Sauce

It's smoking time...

Cooker used

Notes

Log all that deliciousness...

Time	Cooker Target Temp	Cooker Actual Temp	Meat Temp	Weather Temp	Action taken e.g. vents, wood, mop or turn

Results

RATING	1	2	3	4	5	6	7	8	9	10

Notes/serving

Let's get smoking!

Date

The Meat

Cut	Price
Source	Weight
Expiration Date	Fresh/Frozen

Notes

The Prep

Wood Flavour	Soaked/Dry
Wood type	Quantity

Rub/Marinade/Seasoning/Brine

Mop/Paste/Sauce

It's smoking time...

Cooker used

Notes

Log all that deliciousness...

Time	Cooker Target Temp	Cooker Actual Temp	Meat Temp	Weather Temp	Action taken e.g. vents, wood, mop or turn

Results

RATING	1	2	3	4	5	6	7	8	9	10

Notes/serving

Let's get smoking!

Date

The Meat

Cut	Price
Source	Weight
Expiration Date	Fresh/Frozen

Notes

The Prep

Wood Flavour	Soaked/Dry
Wood type	Quantity

Rub/Marinade/Seasoning/Brine

Mop/Paste/Sauce

It's smoking time...

Cooker used

Notes

Log all that deliciousness...

Time	Cooker Target Temp	Cooker Actual Temp	Meat Temp	Weather Temp	Action taken e.g. vents, wood, mop or turn

Results

| RATING | 1 | 2 | 3 | 4 | 5 | 6 | 7 | 8 | 9 | 10 |

Notes/serving

Let's get smoking!

Date

The Meat

Cut		Price	
Source		Weight	
Expiration Date		Fresh/Frozen	

Notes

The Prep

Wood Flavour		Soaked/Dry	
Wood type		Quantity	

Rub/Marinade/Seasoning/Brine

Mop/Paste/Sauce

It's smoking time...

Cooker used

Notes

Log all that deliciousness...

Time	Cooker Target Temp	Cooker Actual Temp	Meat Temp	Weather Temp	Action taken e.g. vents, wood, mop or turn

Results

RATING	1	2	3	4	5	6	7	8	9	10

Notes/serving

Let's get smoking!

Date

The Meat

Cut	Price
Source	Weight
Expiration Date	Fresh/Frozen

Notes

The Prep

Wood Flavour	Soaked/Dry
Wood type	Quantity

Rub/Marinade/Seasoning/Brine

Mop/Paste/Sauce

It's smoking time...

Cooker used

Notes

Log all that deliciousness...

Time	Cooker Target Temp	Cooker Actual Temp	Meat Temp	Weather Temp	Action taken e.g. vents, wood, mop or turn

Results

RATING 1 2 3 4 5 6 7 8 9 10

Notes/serving

Let's get smoking!

Date

The Meat

Cut	Price
Source	Weight
Expiration Date	Fresh/Frozen

Notes

The Prep

Wood Flavour	Soaked/Dry
Wood type	Quantity

Rub/Marinade/Seasoning/Brine

Mop/Paste/Sauce

It's smoking time...

Cooker used

Notes

Log all that deliciousness...

Time	Cooker Target Temp	Cooker Actual Temp	Meat Temp	Weather Temp	Action taken e.g. vents, wood, mop or turn

Results

RATING   1   2   3   4   5   6   7   8   9   10

Notes/serving

Let's get smoking!

Date

The Meat

Cut		Price	
Source		Weight	
Expiration Date		Fresh/Frozen	

Notes

The Prep

Wood Flavour		Soaked/Dry	
Wood type		Quantity	

Rub/Marinade/Seasoning/Brine

Mop/Paste/Sauce

It's smoking time...

Cooker used

Notes

Log all that deliciousness...

Time	Cooker Target Temp	Cooker Actual Temp	Meat Temp	Weather Temp	Action taken e.g. vents, wood, mop or turn

Results

RATING	1	2	3	4	5	6	7	8	9	10

Notes/serving

Let's get smoking!

Date

The Meat

Cut	Price
Source	Weight
Expiration Date	Fresh/Frozen

Notes

The Prep

Wood Flavour	Soaked/Dry
Wood type	Quantity

Rub/Marinade/Seasoning/Brine

Mop/Paste/Sauce

It's smoking time...

Cooker used

Notes

Log all that deliciousness...

Time	Cooker Target Temp	Cooker Actual Temp	Meat Temp	Weather Temp	Action taken e.g. vents, wood, mop or turn

Results

RATING	1	2	3	4	5	6	7	8	9	10

Notes/serving

Let's get smoking!

Date

The Meat

Cut		Price	
Source		Weight	
Expiration Date		Fresh/Frozen	

Notes

The Prep

Wood Flavour		Soaked/Dry	
Wood type		Quantity	

Rub/Marinade/Seasoning/Brine

Mop/Paste/Sauce

It's smoking time...

Cooker used

Notes

Log all that deliciousness...

Time	Cooker Target Temp	Cooker Actual Temp	Meat Temp	Weather Temp	Action taken e.g. vents, wood, mop or turn

Results

RATING   1   2   3   4   5   6   7   8   9   10

Notes/serving

Let's get smoking!

Date

The Meat

Cut	Price
Source	Weight
Expiration Date	Fresh/Frozen
Notes	

The Prep

Wood Flavour	Soaked/Dry
Wood type	Quantity
Rub/Marinade/Seasoning/Brine	
Mop/Paste/Sauce	

It's smoking time...

Cooker used
Notes

Log all that deliciousness...

Time	Cooker Target Temp	Cooker Actual Temp	Meat Temp	Weather Temp	Action taken e.g. vents, wood, mop or turn

Results

RATING	1	2	3	4	5	6	7	8	9	10

Notes/serving

Let's get smoking!

Date

The Meat

Cut		Price	
Source		Weight	
Expiration Date		Fresh/Frozen	

Notes

The Prep

Wood Flavour		Soaked/Dry	
Wood type		Quantity	

Rub/Marinade/Seasoning/Brine

Mop/Paste/Sauce

It's smoking time...

Cooker used

Notes

Log all that deliciousness...

Time	Cooker Target Temp	Cooker Actual Temp	Meat Temp	Weather Temp	Action taken e.g. vents, wood, mop or turn

Results

RATING	1	2	3	4	5	6	7	8	9	10

Notes/serving

Let's get smoking!

Date

The Meat

Cut	Price
Source	Weight
Expiration Date	Fresh/Frozen

Notes

The Prep

Wood Flavour	Soaked/Dry
Wood type	Quantity

Rub/Marinade/Seasoning/Brine

Mop/Paste/Sauce

It's smoking time...

Cooker used

Notes

Log all that deliciousness...

Time	Cooker Target Temp	Cooker Actual Temp	Meat Temp	Weather Temp	Action taken e.g. vents, wood, mop or turn

Results

RATING	1	2	3	4	5	6	7	8	9	10

Notes/serving

Let's get smoking!

Date

The Meat

Cut	Price
Source	Weight
Expiration Date	Fresh/Frozen
Notes	

The Prep

Wood Flavour	Soaked/Dry
Wood type	Quantity
Rub/Marinade/Seasoning/Brine	
Mop/Paste/Sauce	

It's smoking time...

Cooker used
Notes

Log all that deliciousness...

Time	Cooker Target Temp	Cooker Actual Temp	Meat Temp	Weather Temp	Action taken e.g. vents, wood, mop or turn

Results

RATING	1	2	3	4	5	6	7	8	9	10

Notes/serving

Let's get smoking!

Date

The Meat

Cut	Price
Source	Weight
Expiration Date	Fresh/Frozen

Notes

The Prep

Wood Flavour	Soaked/Dry
Wood type	Quantity

Rub/Marinade/Seasoning/Brine

Mop/Paste/Sauce

It's smoking time...

Cooker used

Notes

Log all that deliciousness...

Time	Cooker Target Temp	Cooker Actual Temp	Meat Temp	Weather Temp	Action taken e.g. vents, wood, mop or turn

Results

RATING	1	2	3	4	5	6	7	8	9	10

Notes/serving

Let's get smoking!

Date

The Meat

Cut		Price	
Source		Weight	
Expiration Date		Fresh/Frozen	

Notes

The Prep

Wood Flavour		Soaked/Dry	
Wood type		Quantity	

Rub/Marinade/Seasoning/Brine

Mop/Paste/Sauce

It's smoking time...

Cooker used

Notes

Log all that deliciousness...

Time	Cooker Target Temp	Cooker Actual Temp	Meat Temp	Weather Temp	Action taken e.g. vents, wood, mop or turn

Results

RATING	1	2	3	4	5	6	7	8	9	10

Notes/serving

Let's get smoking!

Date

The Meat

Cut	Price
Source	Weight
Expiration Date	Fresh/Frozen

Notes

The Prep

Wood Flavour	Soaked/Dry
Wood type	Quantity

Rub/Marinade/Seasoning/Brine

Mop/Paste/Sauce

It's smoking time...

Cooker used

Notes

Log all that deliciousness...

Time	Cooker Target Temp	Cooker Actual Temp	Meat Temp	Weather Temp	Action taken e.g. vents, wood, mop or turn

Results

RATING 1 2 3 4 5 6 7 8 9 10

Notes/serving

Let's get smoking!

Date

The Meat

Cut	Price
Source	Weight
Expiration Date	Fresh/Frozen
Notes	

The Prep

Wood Flavour	Soaked/Dry
Wood type	Quantity
Rub/Marinade/Seasoning/Brine	
Mop/Paste/Sauce	

It's smoking time...

Cooker used
Notes

Log all that deliciousness...

Time	Cooker Target Temp	Cooker Actual Temp	Meat Temp	Weather Temp	Action taken e.g. vents, wood, mop or turn

Results

RATING	1 2 3 4 5 6 7 8 9 10
Notes/serving	

Let's get smoking!

Date

The Meat

Cut		Price	
Source		Weight	
Expiration Date		Fresh/Frozen	
Notes			

The Prep

Wood Flavour		Soaked/Dry	
Wood type		Quantity	
Rub/Marinade/Seasoning/Brine			
Mop/Paste/Sauce			

It's smoking time...

Cooker used
Notes

Log all that deliciousness...

Time	Cooker Target Temp	Cooker Actual Temp	Meat Temp	Weather Temp	Action taken e.g. vents, wood, mop or turn

Results

RATING	1	2	3	4	5	6	7	8	9	10

Notes/serving

Let's get smoking!

Date

The Meat

Cut	Price
Source	Weight
Expiration Date	Fresh/Frozen
Notes	

The Prep

Wood Flavour	Soaked/Dry
Wood type	Quantity
Rub/Marinade/Seasoning/Brine	
Mop/Paste/Sauce	

It's smoking time...

Cooker used
Notes

Log all that deliciousness...

Time	Cooker Target Temp	Cooker Actual Temp	Meat Temp	Weather Temp	Action taken e.g. vents, wood, mop or turn

Results

RATING   1   2   3   4   5   6   7   8   9   10

Notes/serving

Let's get smoking!

Date

The Meat

Cut	Price
Source	Weight
Expiration Date	Fresh/Frozen

Notes

The Prep

Wood Flavour	Soaked/Dry
Wood type	Quantity

Rub/Marinade/Seasoning/Brine

Mop/Paste/Sauce

It's smoking time...

Cooker used

Notes

Log all that deliciousness...

Time	Cooker Target Temp	Cooker Actual Temp	Meat Temp	Weather Temp	Action taken e.g. vents, wood, mop or turn

Results

RATING   1   2   3   4   5   6   7   8   9   10

Notes/serving

Let's get smoking!

Date

The Meat

Cut	Price
Source	Weight
Expiration Date	Fresh/Frozen

Notes

The Prep

Wood Flavour	Soaked/Dry
Wood type	Quantity

Rub/Marinade/Seasoning/Brine

Mop/Paste/Sauce

It's smoking time...

Cooker used

Notes

Log all that deliciousness...

Time	Cooker Target Temp	Cooker Actual Temp	Meat Temp	Weather Temp	Action taken e.g. vents, wood, mop or turn

Results

RATING 1   2   3   4   5   6   7   8   9   10

Notes/serving

Let's get smoking!

Date

The Meat

Cut	Price
Source	Weight
Expiration Date	Fresh/Frozen

Notes

The Prep

Wood Flavour	Soaked/Dry
Wood type	Quantity

Rub/Marinade/Seasoning/Brine

Mop/Paste/Sauce

It's smoking time...

Cooker used

Notes

Log all that deliciousness...

Time	Cooker Target Temp	Cooker Actual Temp	Meat Temp	Weather Temp	Action taken e.g. vents, wood, mop or turn

Results

RATING	1 2 3 4 5 6 7 8 9 10

Notes/serving

Let's get smoking!

Date

The Meat

Cut		Price	
Source		Weight	
Expiration Date		Fresh/Frozen	
Notes			

The Prep

Wood Flavour		Soaked/Dry	
Wood type		Quantity	
Rub/Marinade/Seasoning/Brine			
Mop/Paste/Sauce			

It's smoking time...

Cooker used
Notes

Log all that deliciousness...

Time	Cooker Target Temp	Cooker Actual Temp	Meat Temp	Weather Temp	Action taken e.g. vents, wood, mop or turn

Results

RATING	1	2	3	4	5	6	7	8	9	10

Notes/serving

Let's get smoking!

Date

The Meat

Cut	Price
Source	Weight
Expiration Date	Fresh/Frozen
Notes	

The Prep

Wood Flavour	Soaked/Dry
Wood type	Quantity
Rub/Marinade/Seasoning/Brine	
Mop/Paste/Sauce	

It's smoking time...

Cooker used
Notes

Log all that deliciousness...

Time	Cooker Target Temp	Cooker Actual Temp	Meat Temp	Weather Temp	Action taken e.g. vents, wood, mop or turn

Results

RATING 1 2 3 4 5 6 7 8 9 10

Notes/serving

Let's get smoking!

Date

The Meat

Cut	Price
Source	Weight
Expiration Date	Fresh/Frozen
Notes	

The Prep

Wood Flavour	Soaked/Dry
Wood type	Quantity
Rub/Marinade/Seasoning/Brine	
Mop/Paste/Sauce	

It's smoking time...

Cooker used
Notes

Log all that deliciousness...

Time	Cooker Target Temp	Cooker Actual Temp	Meat Temp	Weather Temp	Action taken e.g. vents, wood, mop or turn

Results

RATING   1   2   3   4   5   6   7   8   9   10

Notes/serving

Let's get smoking!

Date

The Meat

Cut	Price
Source	Weight
Expiration Date	Fresh/Frozen

Notes

The Prep

Wood Flavour	Soaked/Dry
Wood type	Quantity

Rub/Marinade/Seasoning/Brine

Mop/Paste/Sauce

It's smoking time...

Cooker used

Notes

Log all that deliciousness...

Time	Cooker Target Temp	Cooker Actual Temp	Meat Temp	Weather Temp	Action taken e.g. vents, wood, mop or turn

Results

RATING	1	2	3	4	5	6	7	8	9	10

Notes/serving

Let's get smoking!

Date

The Meat

Cut	Price
Source	Weight
Expiration Date	Fresh/Frozen

Notes

The Prep

Wood Flavour	Soaked/Dry
Wood type	Quantity

Rub/Marinade/Seasoning/Brine

Mop/Paste/Sauce

It's smoking time...

Cooker used

Notes

Log all that deliciousness...

Time	Cooker Target Temp	Cooker Actual Temp	Meat Temp	Weather Temp	Action taken e.g. vents, wood, mop or turn

Results

RATING	1	2	3	4	5	6	7	8	9	10

Notes/serving

Let's get smoking!

Date

The Meat

Cut	Price
Source	Weight
Expiration Date	Fresh/Frozen

Notes

The Prep

Wood Flavour	Soaked/Dry
Wood type	Quantity

Rub/Marinade/Seasoning/Brine

Mop/Paste/Sauce

It's smoking time...

Cooker used

Notes

Log all that deliciousness...

Time	Cooker Target Temp	Cooker Actual Temp	Meat Temp	Weather Temp	Action taken e.g. vents, wood, mop or turn

Results

RATING 1 2 3 4 5 6 7 8 9 10

Notes/serving

Let's get smoking!

Date

The Meat

Cut	Price
Source	Weight
Expiration Date	Fresh/Frozen

Notes

The Prep

Wood Flavour	Soaked/Dry
Wood type	Quantity

Rub/Marinade/Seasoning/Brine

Mop/Paste/Sauce

It's smoking time...

Cooker used

Notes

Log all that deliciousness...

Time	Cooker Target Temp	Cooker Actual Temp	Meat Temp	Weather Temp	Action taken e.g. vents, wood, mop or turn

Results

RATING   1   2   3   4   5   6   7   8   9   10

Notes/serving

Let's get smoking!

Date

The Meat

Cut	Price
Source	Weight
Expiration Date	Fresh/Frozen

Notes

The Prep

Wood Flavour	Soaked/Dry
Wood type	Quantity

Rub/Marinade/Seasoning/Brine

Mop/Paste/Sauce

It's smoking time...

Cooker used

Notes

Log all that deliciousness...

Time	Cooker Target Temp	Cooker Actual Temp	Meat Temp	Weather Temp	Action taken e.g. vents, wood, mop or turn

Results

RATING	1	2	3	4	5	6	7	8	9	10

Notes/serving

Let's get smoking!

Date

The Meat

Cut	Price
Source	Weight
Expiration Date	Fresh/Frozen

Notes

The Prep

Wood Flavour	Soaked/Dry
Wood type	Quantity

Rub/Marinade/Seasoning/Brine

Mop/Paste/Sauce

It's smoking time...

Cooker used

Notes

Log all that deliciousness...

Time	Cooker Target Temp	Cooker Actual Temp	Meat Temp	Weather Temp	Action taken e.g. vents, wood, mop or turn

Results

RATING	1 2 3 4 5 6 7 8 9 10

Notes/serving

Let's get smoking!

Date

The Meat

Cut	Price
Source	Weight
Expiration Date	Fresh/Frozen

Notes

The Prep

Wood Flavour	Soaked/Dry
Wood type	Quantity

Rub/Marinade/Seasoning/Brine

Mop/Paste/Sauce

It's smoking time...

Cooker used

Notes

Log all that deliciousness...

Time	Cooker Target Temp	Cooker Actual Temp	Meat Temp	Weather Temp	Action taken e.g. vents, wood, mop or turn

Results

RATING	1	2	3	4	5	6	7	8	9	10

Notes/serving

Let's get smoking!

Date

The Meat

Cut	Price
Source	Weight
Expiration Date	Fresh/Frozen

Notes

The Prep

Wood Flavour	Soaked/Dry
Wood type	Quantity

Rub/Marinade/Seasoning/Brine

Mop/Paste/Sauce

It's smoking time...

Cooker used

Notes

Log all that deliciousness...

Time	Cooker Target Temp	Cooker Actual Temp	Meat Temp	Weather Temp	Action taken e.g. vents, wood, mop or turn

Results

RATING	1	2	3	4	5	6	7	8	9	10

Notes/serving

Let's get smoking!

Date

The Meat

Cut	Price
Source	Weight
Expiration Date	Fresh/Frozen
Notes	

The Prep

Wood Flavour	Soaked/Dry
Wood type	Quantity
Rub/Marinade/Seasoning/Brine	
Mop/Paste/Sauce	

It's smoking time...

Cooker used
Notes

Log all that deliciousness...

Time	Cooker Target Temp	Cooker Actual Temp	Meat Temp	Weather Temp	Action taken e.g. vents, wood, mop or turn

Results

| RATING | 1 | 2 | 3 | 4 | 5 | 6 | 7 | 8 | 9 | 10 |

Notes/serving

Let's get smoking!

Date

The Meat

Cut	Price
Source	Weight
Expiration Date	Fresh/Frozen
Notes	

The Prep

Wood Flavour	Soaked/Dry
Wood type	Quantity
Rub/Marinade/Seasoning/Brine	
Mop/Paste/Sauce	

It's smoking time...

Cooker used
Notes

Log all that deliciousness...

Time	Cooker Target Temp	Cooker Actual Temp	Meat Temp	Weather Temp	Action taken e.g. vents, wood, mop or turn

Results

RATING	1	2	3	4	5	6	7	8	9	10

Notes/serving

Let's get smoking!

Date

The Meat

Cut	Price
Source	Weight
Expiration Date	Fresh/Frozen

Notes

The Prep

Wood Flavour	Soaked/Dry
Wood type	Quantity

Rub/Marinade/Seasoning/Brine

Mop/Paste/Sauce

It's smoking time...

Cooker used

Notes

Log all that deliciousness...

Time	Cooker Target Temp	Cooker Actual Temp	Meat Temp	Weather Temp	Action taken e.g. vents, wood, mop or turn

Results

RATING   1   2   3   4   5   6   7   8   9   10

Notes/serving

Let's get smoking!

Date

The Meat

Cut	Price
Source	Weight
Expiration Date	Fresh/Frozen

Notes

The Prep

Wood Flavour	Soaked/Dry
Wood type	Quantity

Rub/Marinade/Seasoning/Brine

Mop/Paste/Sauce

It's smoking time...

Cooker used

Notes

Log all that deliciousness...

Time	Cooker Target Temp	Cooker Actual Temp	Meat Temp	Weather Temp	Action taken e.g. vents, wood, mop or turn

Results

RATING   1   2   3   4   5   6   7   8   9   10

Notes/serving

Let's get smoking!

Date

The Meat

Cut	Price
Source	Weight
Expiration Date	Fresh/Frozen

Notes

The Prep

Wood Flavour	Soaked/Dry
Wood type	Quantity

Rub/Marinade/Seasoning/Brine

Mop/Paste/Sauce

It's smoking time...

Cooker used

Notes

Log all that deliciousness...

Time	Cooker Target Temp	Cooker Actual Temp	Meat Temp	Weather Temp	Action taken e.g. vents, wood, mop or turn

Results

RATING	1	2	3	4	5	6	7	8	9	10

Notes/serving

Let's get smoking!

Date

The Meat

Cut	Price
Source	Weight
Expiration Date	Fresh/Frozen

Notes

The Prep

Wood Flavour	Soaked/Dry
Wood type	Quantity

Rub/Marinade/Seasoning/Brine

Mop/Paste/Sauce

It's smoking time...

Cooker used

Notes

Log all that deliciousness...

Time	Cooker Target Temp	Cooker Actual Temp	Meat Temp	Weather Temp	Action taken e.g. vents, wood, mop or turn

Results

RATING 1 2 3 4 5 6 7 8 9 10

Notes/serving

Let's get smoking!

Date

The Meat

Cut	Price
Source	Weight
Expiration Date	Fresh/Frozen

Notes

The Prep

Wood Flavour	Soaked/Dry
Wood type	Quantity

Rub/Marinade/Seasoning/Brine

Mop/Paste/Sauce

It's smoking time...

Cooker used

Notes

Log all that deliciousness...

Time	Cooker Target Temp	Cooker Actual Temp	Meat Temp	Weather Temp	Action taken e.g. vents, wood, mop or turn

Results

RATING 1 2 3 4 5 6 7 8 9 10

Notes/serving

Let's get smoking!

Date

The Meat

Cut	Price
Source	Weight
Expiration Date	Fresh/Frozen

Notes

The Prep

Wood Flavour	Soaked/Dry
Wood type	Quantity

Rub/Marinade/Seasoning/Brine

Mop/Paste/Sauce

It's smoking time...

Cooker used

Notes

www.ingramcontent.com/pod-product-compliance
Lightning Source LLC
Chambersburg PA
CBHW080600030426
42336CB00019B/3266

* 9 7 8 1 6 4 9 4 4 1 3 0 0 *